GAO

Report to the Subcommittee on Oversight of Government Management, the Federal Workforce, and the District of Columbia, Committee on Homeland Security and Governmental Affairs, U.S. Senate

July 2012

WORLD HEALTH ORGANIZATION

I0413287

Reform Agenda Developed, but U.S. Actions to Monitor Progress Could be Enhanced

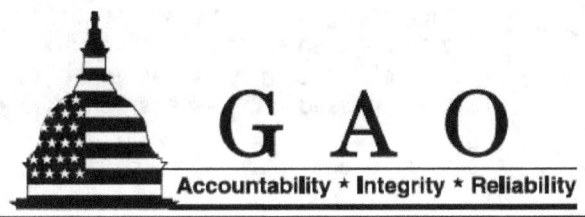

GAO

Accountability ★ Integrity ★ Reliability

GAO-12-722

G A O
Accountability * Integrity * Reliability

Highlights

Highlights of GAO-12-722, a report to the Subcommittee on Oversight of Government Management, the Federal Workforce, and the District of Columbia, Committee on Homeland Security and Governmental Affairs, U.S. Senate

WORLD HEALTH ORGANIZATION

Reform Agenda Developed, but U.S. Actions to Monitor Progress Could Be Enhanced

Why GAO Did This Study

WHO is the directing and coordinating authority for global health within the United Nations (UN) system. In 2012, member states approved a reform agenda addressing three areas: (1) priority-setting, to refocus its efforts and establish a process to determine priorities; (2) governance, to improve the effectiveness of its governing bodies and strengthen engagement with other stakeholders; and (3) management, including human resources, results-based planning, and accountability. The United States is a key participant in WHO's governing bodies and the largest donor, contributing about $219 million, or 22 percent, to WHO's assessed budget for 2010 and 2011, and more than $475 million, or about 16 percent, to WHO's voluntary budget. As the largest financial contributor to the UN, the United States has advocated for comprehensive management reform throughout the UN system, including WHO. This report examines (1) the steps WHO has taken to develop and implement a reform agenda that aligns with the challenges identified by stakeholders and (2) the input the United States has provided to WHO reforms. GAO analyzed WHO and U.S. government documents and interviewed officials and stakeholders in Washington, D.C., and Geneva, Switzerland.

What GAO Recommends

GAO recommends that the Secretary of State enhance State's guidance on completing its assessment tool for monitoring WHO's progress in implementing transparency and accountability reforms. State generally concurred with GAO's recommendation.

View GAO-12-722. For more information, contact Thomas Melito at (202) 512-9601 or melitot@gao.gov.

What GAO Found

In May 2012, 194 member states approved components of the World Health Organization's (WHO) reform agenda, encompassing three broad areas—priority-setting, governance, and management reforms—that generally address the challenges identified by stakeholders. According to WHO officials, member state representatives, and other stakeholders, some of the challenges facing WHO include its (1) lack of clear organizational priorities; (2) lack of predictable and flexible financing; and (3) highly decentralized organizational structure. In developing its reform agenda, WHO consulted with member states, employees, and other parties to gather their views and feedback. In addition, WHO has commissioned three ongoing evaluations to provide input into the reform process. The first stage of one of the planned evaluations was conducted by WHO's External Auditor, which concluded in March 2012 that WHO's reform proposals are comprehensive in addressing challenges faced by the organization. WHO continues to consult with member states on priority-setting and governance proposals, which generally require extensive deliberation and consensus from member states. In November 2011, the WHO Executive Board approved WHO's management reform proposals in several areas, and requested further development of proposals in other areas. In May 2012, WHO developed a high-level implementation and monitoring framework that includes reform objectives, selected activities, 1-year and 3-year milestones, and intended impacts. Certain factors could impede WHO's ability to successfully implement its reform proposals, including the availability of sufficient financial and technical resources and the level of sustained support from internal and external stakeholders.

The United States has provided input into WHO's reform agenda, particularly in the areas of transparency and accountability, but the Department of State's (State) tool for assessing progress in the area of management reform could be enhanced. On priority-setting, the United States has advocated for WHO to maintain its focus on certain functions such as setting regulations and standards for international health. In consultations on governance, the U.S. delegation to WHO has commented on a range of proposals WHO has put forth, including those on engagement with other global health stakeholders. On management reforms, the United States has supported an agenda for greater transparency and accountability. The U.S. delegation has advocated for a number of reforms to improve WHO's internal and external oversight mechanisms and supported reforms in budgeting, planning, and human resources. Additionally, State has established an assessment tool to measure progress on transparency and accountability mechanisms, which is a useful tool for guiding U.S. priorities and engagement with WHO, and could be helpful for monitoring WHO's progress in implementing certain management reforms. However, we found weaknesses in State's assessment tool, including an unclear basis for State's determinations on certain elements in its assessment of WHO, as well as a lack of clarity in the definitions used in the assessment. According to State officials, State provides guidance to officials completing these assessments but acknowledged that the process does not fully mitigate risks to data reliability.

_____ United States Government Accountability Office

Contents

Figures

Abbreviations

CDC	Centers for Disease Control and Prevention
HHS	Department of Health and Human Services
JIU	United Nations Joint Inspection Unit
NIH	National Institutes of Health
PAHO	Pan American Health Organization
State	Department of State
UN	United Nations
UNTAI	United Nations Transparency and Accountability Initiative
USAID	U.S. Agency for International Development
USUN-Geneva	U.S. Mission to the United Nations in Geneva
WHO	World Health Organization

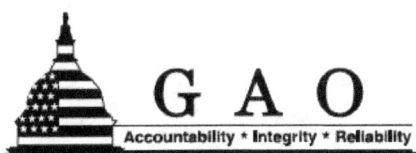

United States Government Accountability Office
Washington, DC 20548

July 23, 2012

The Honorable Daniel K. Akaka
Chairman
The Honorable Ron Johnson
Ranking Member
Subcommittee on Oversight of Government Management,
    the Federal Workforce, and the District of Columbia
Committee on Homeland Security and Governmental Affairs
United States Senate

The World Health Organization (WHO) is the directing and coordinating authority for global health within the United Nations (UN) system. In this capacity, WHO is responsible for providing leadership on important global health matters such as setting standards and guidelines for international health, providing technical support on public health to countries, and monitoring and assessing global health trends. The United States is a key participant in WHO's governing bodies and the largest donor to WHO, contributing about $219 million, or 22 percent, to WHO's regular, assessed budget for 2010 and 2011,[1] as well as more than $475 million, or about 16 percent, to WHO's voluntary budget.[2]

In January 2010, WHO's Director-General initiated discussions with member states on the predictability and flexibility of WHO's financing and how its funding could be better aligned with its priorities. Through a series of continued consultations and deliberations, member states and other stakeholders raised a wide range of other concerns, including questions about WHO's core business in an increasingly complex and changing global health environment, its role in global health governance, and its organizational effectiveness and efficiency. Accordingly, WHO developed an agenda that expanded beyond financing concerns to address three broad areas of reform: (1) priority-setting, to refocus its efforts on what it can do best and establish a process to determine its priorities; (2)

---

[1]WHO's biennial budget is based on a 2-year budget period.

[2]WHO's budget is comprised of assessed contributions from member states, which are based on the assessed dues for each country, as well as voluntary contributions provided by member states and other entities on a voluntary basis. Voluntary contributions are often specified for certain issues such as particular diseases.

governance, to improve the effectiveness of its governing bodies and strengthen its engagement with other global health stakeholders, including nongovernmental organizations and private industry; and (3) management, to address issues such as human resources, results-based planning, and accountability. Implementation of WHO's reform agenda remains in the early stages.

As the largest financial contributor to the UN, the United States holds a strong interest in the progress of UN reform initiatives and has advocated for comprehensive management reform at UN agencies, including WHO. Accordingly, the U.S. Department of State (State) developed the United Nations Transparency and Accountability Initiative (UNTAI), to promote greater efficiency, effectiveness, transparency, and accountability among UN agencies, including WHO. As part of this initiative, State developed an assessment tool that it uses to conduct annual assessments to measure UN agency performance and progress in eight goals related to transparency and accountability. Additionally, the U.S. Department of Health and Human Services (HHS) is responsible for coordinating U.S. government input into the policies and decisions of health-related international organizations, including WHO.

As part of our continuing work on UN management reform,[3] this report examines (1) the steps WHO has taken to develop and implement a reform agenda that aligns with the challenges identified by the organization, its member states, and other stakeholders; and (2) the input the United States has provided to WHO reforms.

To address these objectives, we reviewed relevant WHO documents and U.S. government data and documents including position papers, talking points, and speeches, and met with officials from State and HHS, including the Centers for Disease Control and Prevention (CDC), and the U.S. Agency for International Development (USAID). We also assessed the UNTAI assessment tool, which State uses to measure the performance and progress of UN agencies, including WHO, on transparency and accountability. In Washington, D.C., and during fieldwork in Geneva, Switzerland, in December 2011, we interviewed WHO officials and officials at the U.S. Mission to the UN in Geneva (USUN-Geneva), as well as representatives from 15 other member state

---

[3]See Related GAO Products at the end of this report.

missions, and a range of other global health stakeholders. In addition, we held telephone or in-person meetings with officials from each of the six WHO regional offices as well as five country offices. We conducted this performance audit from August 2011 to July 2012 in accordance with generally accepted government auditing standards. Those standards require that we plan and perform the audit to obtain sufficient, appropriate evidence to provide a reasonable basis for our findings and conclusions based on our audit objectives. We believe the evidence obtained provides a reasonable basis for our findings and conclusions based on our audit objectives. (see app. I for further details on our objectives, scope, and methodology).

To improve U.S. assessment of WHO reform, we are recommending that the Secretary of State enhance its guidance on completing State's assessment tool for monitoring WHO's progress in implementing transparency and accountability reforms. We requested comments on a draft of this report from the Departments of State and HHS, USAID, and WHO. State and WHO provided written comments that are reprinted in appendixes III and IV of this report. State generally endorsed the main findings and conclusions of our report. State agreed that its process for conducting its assessment for monitoring progress in implementing transparency and accountability reforms could be strengthened and accepted GAO's recommendation to revise its guidance for completing these assessments. State also offered some clarifications and additional context regarding its assessments. WHO also concurred with the main conclusions of our report and noted that the conclusions broadly converge with those of the evaluation conducted by WHO's External Auditor. In addition, State, HHS, USAID, and WHO provided technical comments that we incorporated into this report, as appropriate.

Background

WHO Structure and Governance

WHO was established in 1948 as the directing and coordinating authority on global health within the UN system. WHO's stated mission is the attainment by all peoples of the highest possible level of health. WHO experts produce health guidelines and standards and assist countries in addressing public health issues. WHO membership is comprised of 194 countries and associate members that meet every year at the World

Health Assembly, WHO's supreme governing body, to set policy and approve the budget.[4] The work of the World Health Assembly is supported by an Executive Board that meets at least twice a year and is composed of 34 members who are technically qualified in the field of health and who hold 3-year terms. The main functions of the Executive Board are to carry out the decisions and policies of the World Health Assembly, provide advice, and facilitate its work. WHO is headed by the Director-General, who is appointed by the World Health Assembly every 5 years.[5] WHO is staffed by approximately 8,000 health and other experts and support staff, working at WHO headquarters in Geneva, Switzerland; six regional offices;[6] and 147 country offices. Each WHO region has a regional committee comprised of representatives from the region's member states, which formulates policies and programs and supervises the work of the regional offices. The regional committees also provide input into global policy and program development through regional consultations. WHO country offices support host countries in policy making, capacity building, and knowledge management, among other things, in the public health sector. Figure 1 shows the WHO regions, their program budgets for 2010 through 2011, and staffing levels.

[4]"Associate members" refers to territories that are not responsible for the conduct of their international relations that may be admitted to WHO upon application made on their behalf by the member or other authority responsible for their international relations.

[5]The current Director-General was appointed by the World Health Assembly in November 2006, and appointed for a second term at the 65th World Health Assembly in May 2012. Her current term runs through June 2017.

[6]WHO regional offices are located in Brazzaville, Congo (African region); Cairo, Egypt (Eastern Mediterranean region); Copenhagen, Denmark (European region); Manila, Philippines (Western Pacific region); New Delhi, India (South-East Asian region); and Washington, D.C. (region of the Americas). The Pan American Health Organization (PAHO), the specialized health agency of the Inter-American System, also serves as the WHO regional office for the Americas as part of the UN system.

Figure 1: WHO Regions, Budgets, and Staffing Levels

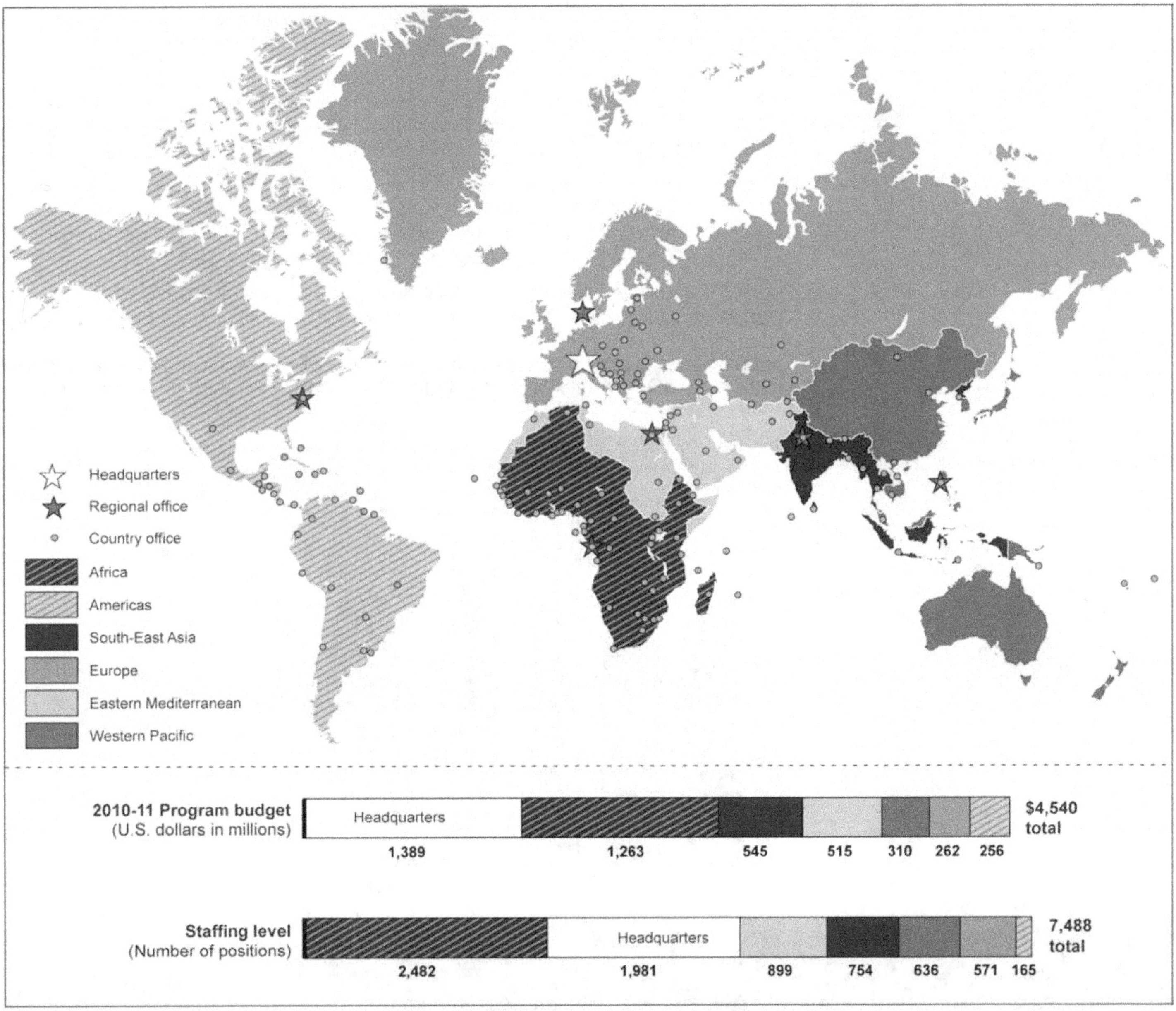

Legend:
- ☆ Headquarters
- ★ Regional office
- ○ Country office
- Africa
- Americas
- South-East Asia
- Europe
- Eastern Mediterranean
- Western Pacific

2010-11 Program budget (U.S. dollars in millions):
Headquarters 1,389 | 1,263 | 545 | 515 | 310 | 262 | 256 — $4,540 total

Staffing level (Number of positions):
2,482 | Headquarters 1,981 | 899 | 754 | 636 | 571 | 165 — 7,488 total

Sources: GAO analysis based on WHO data; Map Resources (map).

Notes: The Pan American Health Organization (PAHO), which serves as the WHO regional office for the Americas, receives funding directly from WHO, in addition to collecting its own assessed and voluntary contributions as a function of its separate role as a public international health organization for the Americas. The budget and staffing figures above indicate the portion of the WHO budget and staff allocated to PAHO. However, PAHO's budget also includes funds collected directly from member states in the Americas.

Staffing data are as of December 31, 2011, and do not include 329 staff who work on WHO special programs and collaborative arrangements.

WHO Budget

WHO's total program budget for the 2010-2011 biennium was about $4.5 billion, with staff costs of more than 50 percent of its budget. For the 2010-2011 program budget, the portion of assessed contributions was about 21 percent of the total (approximately $900 million), while voluntary contributions accounted for about 79 percent of the total (approximately $3.6 billion). Voluntary contributions have increased from about 69 percent in 2004 to 2005 to 79 percent in 2010 to 2011 (see fig. 2).

Figure 2: WHO Biennial Program Budgets, from 2004 through 2011, by Funding Type

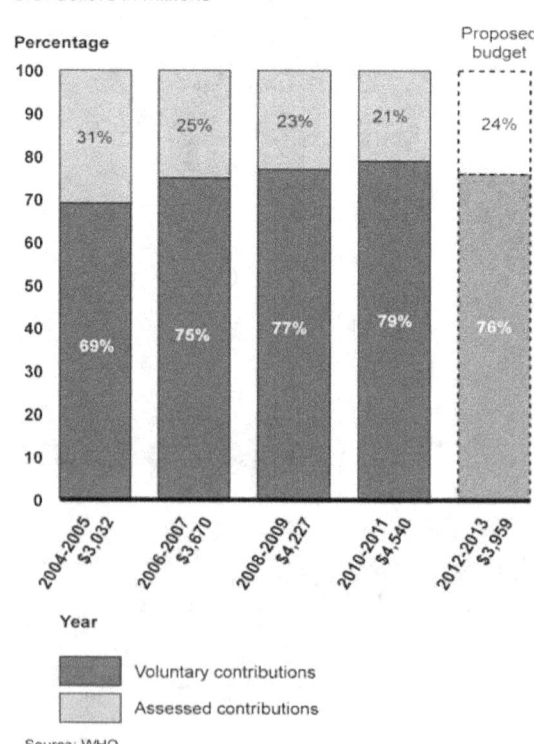

U.S. dollars in millions

Source: WHO.

During the 2010-2011 biennium, the largest annual assessed contributions from member states came from the United States ($219 million), Japan ($135 million), Germany ($77 million), United Kingdom ($62 million), and France ($59 million).[7] While member states are the only entities that provide assessed contributions to WHO's program budget, voluntary contributions come from a diverse group of more than 400 entities, including member states, foundations, nongovernmental organizations, UN agencies, and private sector companies. During the 2010-2011 biennium, the United States was the largest donor of voluntary contributions to the WHO, followed closely by the Bill and Melinda Gates Foundation. During this time period, the top 10 donors to the WHO provided over two-thirds of its total voluntary contributions (see table 1).

Table 1: WHO Voluntary Contributions Received from Top 10 Donors, 2010-2011 Biennium

U.S. dollars in millions

Donor	Voluntary contributions	Percentage of total	Cumulative percentage
United States[a]	$475	15.5	15.5
Bill & Melinda Gates Foundation	467	15.2	30.7
United Kingdom	307	10.0	40.7
Canada	181	5.9	46.5
Rotary International	117	3.8	50.3
Norway	116	3.8	54.1
United Nations Development Program	110	3.6	57.7
The GAVI Alliance[b]	99	3.2	60.9
European Commission	97	3.1	64.1
Australia	96	3.1	67.2
Other	1,007	32.8	100.0
Total WHO voluntary contributions	**$3,069**	**100**	**100**

Source: WHO data.

Notes: Funding data represent actual donor contributions to the WHO.

---

[7]Figures are rounded.

[a]U.S. voluntary contributions are primarily provided by USAID and CDC. According to USAID and CDC officials, for 2010 through 2011, USAID provided about $268 million in voluntary contributions and CDC provided approximately $158 million. In addition, the United States provides additional voluntary funding to WHO through other offices, including State's Bureaus of Population, Refugees, and Migration, and International Security and Nonproliferation; the National Institutes of Health; and the Food and Drug Administration.

[b]The GAVI Alliance was formerly known as the Global Alliance for Vaccines and Immunization. The GAVI Alliance is a public-private partnership focused on saving children's lives and protecting people's health by increasing access to immunization in poor countries.

According to WHO officials, most of WHO's voluntary contributions budget is designated by donors for specific diseases and projects. WHO's financial reporting identifies 13 areas, known as strategic objectives, among which its funding is distributed (see table 2). WHO's program budget for 2010 through 2011 was about $4.5 billion. More than half of that amount was allocated for communicable diseases, HIV/AIDS, tuberculosis, and malaria, and WHO's enabling and support functions.

Table 2: WHO Funding by Strategic Objective, 2010 to 2011

U.S. dollars in millions

Strategic objective	Program budget	Percentage of program budget
Communicable diseases	$1,268	28
HIV/AIDS, tuberculosis, and malaria	634	14
Enabling and support functions	524	12
Health systems and services	474	10
Emergencies and disasters	364	8
Child, adolescent, maternal, sexual and reproductive health, and healthy aging	333	7
WHO leadership, governance, and partnerships	223	5
Risk factors for health	162	4
Chronic noncommunicable conditions	146	3
Nutrition, food safety, and food security	120	3
Medical products and technologies	115	3
Healthier environment	114	3
Social and economic determinants of health	63	1
Total	**$4,540**	**100**

Source: WHO data.

Note: Totals may not add due to rounding.

Origins of WHO Reform

In January 2010, the WHO Director-General convened representatives of member states for a high-level consultation on the predictability and flexibility of WHO's financing, and other global health challenges such as WHO's changing role in the international health arena and WHO priorities. While discussions to reform WHO initially began with a focus on its lack of predictable and flexible financing and the need for better alignment between its objectives and resources, WHO's reform efforts have evolved to address more fundamental questions about its priorities, internal governance, role and engagement with other actors in the global health arena, and the managerial reforms needed to make the organization more effective and accountable. In 2010, WHO became concerned with its financial position, particularly due to increased costs resulting, in part, from a decline in the value of the U.S. dollar. In response, the organization implemented several cost-saving measures, such as reducing travel and publications costs.[8] WHO's financial concerns at the time and the results of two external evaluations of the organization served as additional rationales for WHO to undertake a broad management reform agenda.[9] In May 2011, the World Health Assembly passed a resolution endorsing WHO's overall direction of reform.

U.S. Participation in WHO

The United States is a major participant in WHO's governing bodies, with HHS, State, USAID, and CDC playing key roles in participating in and representing U.S. interests in WHO. The Secretary of HHS leads the U.S. delegation to the World Health Assembly, and the Director of HHS's Office of Global Affairs serves as the U.S. Representative to the WHO Executive Board.[10] HHS is responsible for coordinating U.S. government input into the policies and decisions of health-related international organizations, including WHO. Programmatically, HHS collaborates

---

[8]Due to financial concerns, WHO conducted a staffing review in 2011 that resulted in the abolishment of 200 positions based in Geneva. During this period, 43 positions were created in WHO's administrative and information technology center in Kuala Lumpur, Malaysia, to accommodate functions previously performed in Geneva. WHO expects these decisions to result in long-term cost savings.

[9]Multilateral Organization Performance Assessment Network, *Common Approach: World Health Organization, 2010*, January 2011: and the United Kingdom Department for International Development, *Multilateral Aid Review*, March 2011.

[10]Member states are elected to serve 3-year terms on the Executive Board; the United States is currently serving a 3-year term that runs from 2010 through 2013.

closely with WHO through its agencies and offices, including CDC and the National Institutes of Health (NIH). HHS's efforts in conjunction with WHO occur in areas such as HIV/AIDS, tuberculosis, mental health, malaria, and polio eradication. HHS also participates in the governing bodies of certain regional offices, including the regional offices for the Americas and the Western Pacific.

HHS works closely with State's Bureau of International Organization Affairs, which has responsibility for issues related to budgets, audits, human resources, and financial management. Preparation for the governing body meetings, such as the World Health Assembly, is a process that includes coordination among HHS, State, USAID and other stakeholders throughout the year in the development of U.S. policy positions and programmatic strategies. In addition to governing body meetings, USUN-Geneva leads day-to-day engagement with WHO officials, with support from HHS, CDC, State, and USAID. There are 35 CDC staff assigned to WHO offices throughout the world, including 9 staff at WHO headquarters in Geneva working in areas such as measles, flu, and polio. According to HHS officials, other U.S. agencies also periodically work with WHO on health issues. For example, the Department of Defense works with WHO on health security and disease detection, and in September 2011, WHO and the U.S. government signed a memorandum of understanding regarding cooperation on global health security initiatives. In addition, USAID has several ongoing grants to WHO, including headquarters and the country and regional offices, in areas such as influenza, malaria, maternal and child health, and HIV/AIDS.

U.S. Support for UN Reform

The United States has long supported UN reform initiatives and has advocated for comprehensive management reform at UN agencies, including WHO. In 2005, a number of management reforms were introduced to improve transparency and accountability initiatives at the UN. However, other entities in the UN lagged far behind in improving transparency and accountability, according to the U.S. Mission to the UN and officials from State's Bureau of International Organization Affairs. As a result, in 2007, the United States developed UNTAI to promote more efficiency, effectiveness, transparency, and accountability among UN agencies, including WHO. UNTAI identifies eight goals for which member states can exercise greater oversight and increased transparency and accountability to ensure efficiency and effectiveness. These goals include public access to all relevant documentation related to operations and activities, whistleblower protection policies, financial disclosure programs, an effective ethics office, independence of the respective internal oversight bodies, and adoption of international accounting standards.

As part of this initiative, State conducts regular assessments to measure UN agency performance and progress in the eight goals laid out by UNTAI. The assessment presents information concerning the status of each assessed agency against specific benchmarks established by State. These assessments are intended to help the U.S. government identify weaknesses and prioritize engagement at individual UN agencies. In 2011, State established UNTAI phase 2 and revised the UNTAI goals and benchmarks from UNTAI phase 1. UNTAI phase 1 sought to extend reforms already in place at the UN Secretariat to the rest of the UN system, while UNTAI phase 2 was designed to build on UNTAI's successes and focus on further raising accountability standards for the UN system. For example, UNTAI phase 2 added oversight of procurement because the United States has identified this as a high-risk area. Other changes to the UNTAI assessment tool include enterprise risk management and ethics issues such as nepotism, post-employment restrictions, and conflicts of interest.

WHO Developed a Reform Agenda that Generally Aligns with the Challenges Identified by Stakeholders

WHO developed a reform agenda that generally aligns with the challenges identified by stakeholders. In May 2012, member states approved components of WHO's reform agenda, encompassing three broad areas—priority setting, governance, and management reforms— that generally align with challenges identified by stakeholders. According to WHO officials, member state representatives, and other stakeholders, some of the challenges facing WHO include (1) its lack of clear organizational priorities; (2) lack of predictable and flexible financing; and (3) highly decentralized organizational structure. In developing its reform agenda, WHO consulted with member states, employees, and other parties to gather their views and feedback. In addition, WHO has commissioned three ongoing evaluations to provide input into the reform process. The first stage of one of the planned evaluations, conducted by WHO's External Auditor and completed in March 2012, concluded that WHO's reform proposals are generally comprehensive in addressing challenges raised by member states and other stakeholders.[11] WHO

---

[11]WHO's External Auditor, currently the Comptroller and Auditor General of India, authored the *Evaluation Report of Stage 1 of Reform Proposals of WHO*, 2012.

continues to consult with member states on priority-setting and governance proposals, which may require extensive deliberation and consensus from member states. In November 2011, the WHO Executive Board approved WHO's management reform proposals in several areas, and requested further development of proposals in other areas. In May 2012, WHO developed a high-level implementation and monitoring framework that includes reform objectives, selected reform activities, 1-year and 3-year milestones, and intended results. Certain factors could impede WHO's ability to successfully implement its reform proposals, including the availability of sufficient financial and technical resources and the extent of support from internal and external stakeholders.

WHO's Reform Agenda Covers Three Broad Areas

In May 2012, member states approved components of WHO's reform agenda that encompass three broad areas—priority-setting, governance, and management. In the area of priority-setting, WHO seeks to focus its efforts and narrow the scope of its work to what it can do best. WHO also seeks to improve member states' governance of the organization and strengthen its leadership role in the global health arena. Management proposals include efforts to increase WHO's effectiveness by improving its financing, human resources policies, results-based planning, and accountability and transparency mechanisms. Table 3 outlines WHO's three areas of reform and some of WHO's rationales for the reforms in each area.

Table 3: WHO's Areas of Reform and Rationale for Reform

Area of reform	Rationale for reform
Priority-setting	
• Establishment of organizational priorities	• WHO priority-setting has not been sufficiently selective or strategically focused. As a result, WHO is overcommitted and works in too many global health areas.
Governance	
• Effectiveness of WHO internal governance structures	• WHO's internal governance structures need to have a more strategic and disciplined approach to priority-setting.
	• Oversight of the programmatic and financial aspects of the organization needs to be enhanced.
	• The efficiency and inclusivity of the intergovernmental consensus-building process needs to be enhanced.
	• The duration, timing, and sequencing of the sessions of the WHO governing body meetings are not optimal.
• WHO's engagement with external stakeholders	• WHO's role in global health governance needs to be clarified and strengthened.
	• The global health community has greatly expanded, leading to a number of global health organizations with overlapping roles and responsibilities.

GAO-12-722 World Health Organization

Area of reform	Rationale for reform
Management	
• Alignment of WHO headquarters, regional, and country offices	• WHO has a decentralized organizational structure, and roles and responsibilities of the three levels of the organization need to be better defined. • Programs and offices tend to work independently of one another.
• WHO financing	• WHO faces a misalignment between what its governing bodies approve in terms of strategic direction, the budget for the organization, and the resources available. • Voluntary contributions, which represent the major source of WHO's funding, are often highly specified and not aligned with WHO's program budget. • The current level of assessed contributions is not sufficient to carry out WHO's work. • The cost of WHO's administration is not adequately financed.
• Human resources policies and management	• WHO faces a mismatch between its funding and human resources policies. WHO's human resources policies focus on long-term employment while the organization's funding is largely for short-term projects. • The process of recruiting staff is overly complex and lengthy. • Performance management tools are not sufficiently used to evaluate staff performance.
• Results-based management	• WHO faces challenges in measuring its contributions to health outcomes. • WHO resources, outputs, and outcomes are not clearly linked.
• Accountability and transparency	• WHO audit and oversight system has limited capacity. • WHO lacks timely, validated information about its results and resources to provide to member states and governing bodies. • Enforcement of WHO's current accountability and transparency mechanisms is not robust. • WHO's current policies on conflicts of interest and information disclosure are insufficient to deal with the growing complexities of global health.
• Independent evaluation	• WHO does not have an evaluation policy that has been endorsed by its governing bodies, nor does it routinely make its evaluation reports public. • WHO lacks an established mechanism for oversight of evaluation by the governing bodies.
• Strategic communications	• WHO is unable to project a coherent sense of the organization and its achievements.

Source: GAO summary of WHO information.

WHO Undertook Consultations in Developing a Reform Agenda that Generally Aligns with Challenges Identified by Stakeholders

WHO's reform agenda generally aligns with the challenges identified by WHO officials, member states, and other global health organizations we interviewed. According to WHO officials, member state representatives, and other stakeholders, some of the challenges facing WHO include (1) its lack of clear organizational priorities, (2) lack of predictable and flexible financing, and (3) highly decentralized organizational structure. For example, WHO officials and several global health stakeholders stated that, because most of WHO's funding comprises voluntary contributions specified for certain activities, WHO's ability to allocate resources according to its priorities are limited. WHO officials further commented that, while maternal and child health activities and achieving the health-related UN Millennium Development Goals are priorities for the organization, these areas are generally underfunded because donors specify funding for other program areas. In addition, stakeholders stated that WHO's decentralized organizational structure and autonomous regional offices limit the regional and country offices' accountability to WHO headquarters and the coherence of WHO's efforts.

WHO took a number of steps to consult with member states, employees, and other parties to gather their views and feedback on its reform agenda. These consultations are in accordance with a WHO Executive Board decision in May 2011 to establish a transparent, member-state-driven, and inclusive process of consultation to support the development of its reform agenda and proposals. Accordingly, in a previous GAO report, we reported that early, frequent, and clear, two-way communication of information with employees and stakeholders is considered a good practice when undergoing a major organizational change because it allows stakeholders to provide input and take ownership of the change.[12] Figure 3 provides a timeline of WHO consultations with internal and external stakeholders on its reform agenda.

---

[12]GAO, *Results-Oriented Cultures: Implementation Steps to Assist Mergers and Organizational Transformations*, GAO-03-669 (Washington D.C.: Jul. 2, 2003).

Figure 3: Timeline of WHO Consultations with Internal and External Stakeholders, 2011-2012

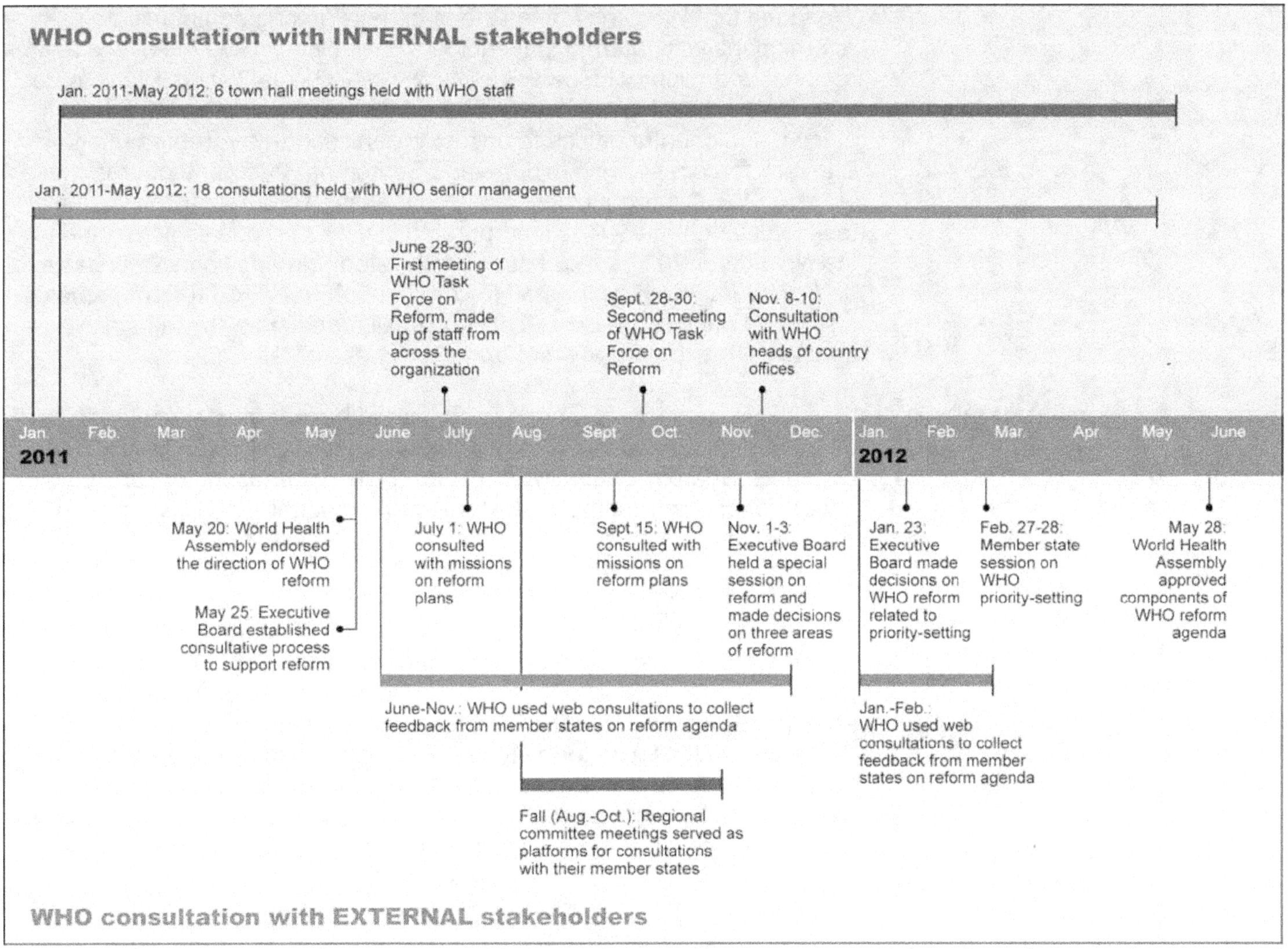

WHO consultation with INTERNAL stakeholders

Jan. 2011-May 2012: 6 town hall meetings held with WHO staff

Jan. 2011-May 2012: 18 consultations held with WHO senior management

June 28-30:
First meeting of
WHO Task
Force on
Reform, made
up of staff from
across the
organization

Sept. 28-30:
Second meeting
of WHO Task
Force on
Reform

Nov. 8-10:
Consultation
with WHO
heads of country
offices

Jan.	Feb.	Mar.	Apr.	May	June	July	Aug.	Sept.	Oct.	Nov.	Dec.	Jan.	Feb.	Mar.	Apr.	May	June
2011												**2012**					

May 20: World Health
Assembly endorsed
the direction of WHO
reform

May 25: Executive
Board established
consultative process
to support reform

July 1: WHO
consulted
with missions
on reform
plans

Sept. 15: WHO
consulted with
missions on
reform plans

Nov. 1-3:
Executive Board
held a special
session on
reform and
made decisions
on three areas
of reform

Jan. 23:
Executive
Board made
decisions on
WHO reform
related to
priority-setting

Feb. 27-28:
Member state
session on
WHO
priority-setting

May 28:
World Health
Assembly
approved
components of
WHO reform
agenda

June-Nov.: WHO used web consultations to collect
feedback from member states on reform agenda

Jan.-Feb.:
WHO used web
consultations to collect
feedback from member
states on reform agenda

Fall (Aug.-Oct.): Regional
committee meetings served as
platforms for consultations
with their member states

WHO consultation with EXTERNAL stakeholders

Source: GAO analysis based on WHO documents

WHO Took Steps to Consult with Internal Stakeholders

We previously reported that a successful organizational transformation must involve employees and their representatives from the beginning to promote their ownership of and investment in the changes occurring in the organization.[13] We also identified the use of employee teams

---

[13]GAO-03-669.

comprising a cross-section of individuals who meet to discuss solutions to specific issues related to organizational change as a promising practice. We found that WHO has taken steps to develop and communicate its reform plans with internal stakeholders, including WHO employees at its regional and country offices. Specifically, WHO established a task force on reform consisting of staff members from headquarters, regional offices, and country offices to ensure organization-wide representation. The task force met twice in June and September 2011 and offered their views on WHO's organizational effectiveness. According to WHO, the task force's feedback was incorporated in WHO proposals presented for the November 2011 special session on reform. In addition, WHO has a dedicated intranet site for staff to comment on the WHO reform process, and WHO officials conducted six town hall meetings with staff since January 2011 to update them on the progress of reform.

WHO Consulted with External Stakeholders through Various Means

WHO used a variety of means to consult with external stakeholders, such as member states, on its reform agenda. As decided at the May 2011 Executive Board session, WHO used private web-based consultations to collect feedback from member states from June through November 2011 and from January through February 2012. WHO also held a 3-day special session of the Executive Board in early November 2011 that was focused on reform. During this session, the WHO Director-General presented WHO's proposals for reform, based on its consultations with member states, as well as a high-level road map for further development of the proposals. The Executive Board made decisions related to the three areas of reform and identified further work to be carried out by the WHO Secretariat. WHO also formally and informally briefed member state missions on its reform proposals and the progress of its reform plans. For example, WHO regional committee meetings that occurred during the fall of 2011 served as platforms for consultations with their member states. According to WHO officials, because reform has generally been a member state-driven process, WHO consultation with nongovernmental organizations and private industry has been more limited than its engagement with member states. However, WHO invited nongovernmental organizations in "official relations" with WHO to submit their comments on its reform agenda.[14] According to WHO officials, it has

---

[14]Nongovernmental organizations in "official relations" with WHO are those organizations that fulfill a set of WHO criteria, such as having an international scope of work and focusing on development work in health and health-related fields. Such organizations have the right to appoint a representative to participate, without right of vote, in WHO meetings.

also convened three informal dialogues with nongovernmental organizations since late 2011.

WHO Commissioned Independent Evaluations to Provide Input to the Reform Process

At the November 2011 special session on reform of the WHO Executive Board, the Board decided to commission three ongoing evaluations to provide input to the reform process. WHO commissioned a two-stage independent evaluation, the first stage of which was conducted by WHO's External Auditor during February and March of 2012. The first stage of the evaluation consisted of a review of the comprehensiveness and adequacy of WHO's reform proposals in finance, human resources, and governance. The External Auditor concluded that WHO's reform proposals were generally comprehensive in addressing concerns raised by member states and other stakeholders. The External Auditor also concluded that WHO followed an inclusive process of deliberations and that it held a wide range of consultations with stakeholders, but that it could have taken additional steps to consult with non member state donors to the organization. The External Auditor recommended that WHO develop plans to prioritize the implementation of its various reform proposals; identify desired outputs, outcomes, and impact; explain the implications of new changes to affected parties; and maintain regular communication with those concerned about the progress of WHO's reform proposals.

Stage two of the evaluation is intended to focus, in particular, on the coherence between and functioning of WHO's three organizational levels—headquarters, regions, and country offices and build on the results of the stage one evaluation. The second stage of the evaluation is also intended to inform reform discussions at the May 2013 World Health Assembly.

In addition, at the request of the WHO Executive Board, the UN Joint Inspection Unit (JIU) is conducting evaluations of WHO's management and administration practices and of the decentralization of WHO offices.[15] The objectives of the JIU reviews are to (1) assess the management and

---

[15]The JIU is the only independent external oversight body of the UN system. It is mandated to conduct evaluations, inspections, and investigations of the UN system, including the specialized agencies. The JIU conducted earlier reviews of WHO's decentralization and management and administration issues. See Joint Inspection Unit, *Decentralization of Organizations within the United Nations system. Part III: The World Health Organization* (JIU/REP/93/2), and Joint Inspection Unit, *Review of Management and Administration in the World Health Organization (WHO)* (JIU/REP/2001/5).

administration practices in WHO and identify areas for improvement; and (2) assess the degree of decentralization and delegation of authority among the WHO headquarters and the regional and country offices, as well as current coordination mechanisms and interactions among the three levels. The results of the JIU reviews are intended to provide input into WHO's decisions on reform. JIU aims to present a report covering its two reviews to the WHO Executive Board in January 2013.

Reform Proposals for Member State Consideration Have Been Developed

In May 2012, member states endorsed components of WHO's reform agenda and requested additional work in certain areas. According to WHO, some of the reform proposals can be implemented relatively quickly while others require more detailed consideration and planning. WHO officials stated that decisions regarding WHO priority-setting and governance are driven by member states and will require their extensive deliberation and consensus. WHO continues to consult with member states on priority-setting and governance proposals, while taking steps to further develop and implement its management reform proposals.

WHO Has Identified Criteria for Establishing Its Priorities

According to WHO officials, the organization is trying to identify criteria for establishing its priorities and determine the global health areas it should focus on and where it is best placed to add value. Since WHO's creation in 1948, many other global health efforts have been initiated; thus, there is a need to ensure that WHO's work is focused on the areas in which it has a "unique function" and comparative advantage. Accordingly, WHO aims to establish a clear set of priorities to guide its resource allocation processes and results-based planning activities. Over 90 member states convened at a session on priority-setting in February 2012. They reached consensus on the criteria and the categories of work that will serve as guidance for the development of WHO's priorities, as laid out in its strategic framework and program budget to be approved by the World Health Assembly in May 2013. Agreed-upon criteria for determining WHO's priorities include current health problems, including the burden of disease at the global, regional, or country levels; the needs of individual countries as articulated in their WHO country strategies; and WHO's comparative advantage, including its capacity to gather and analyze data in response to current and emerging health issues. WHO has also established five technical categories that will provide the primary structure of its program budget and include (1) communicable diseases; (2) noncommunicable diseases; (3) promoting health through the life course; (4) strengthening of health systems; and (5) preparedness, surveillance, and response. WHO will define priorities in each of these categories. However, according to WHO, even when priorities are identified, there is no guarantee that funding for priority areas will be available in part due to the common practice of specifying voluntary funds for particular activities.

WHO Has Developed Some Governance Proposals, although Some Areas Require Further Development, Consultation, and Member State Consensus

WHO has developed proposals for some of its governance reforms; however, other areas will require further development, consultation, and member state consensus. Proposals to improve WHO's governance are two-fold and entail (1) improving the effectiveness of WHO's governing bodies, including its Executive Board, World Health Assembly, and regional committees; and (2) strengthening WHO's leadership role in the global health arena. According to WHO, the Executive Board is currently prevented from fully exercising its oversight and executive role due to the demands it faces in preparing the agenda and work of the World Health Assembly. According to WHO, the number of agenda items before the World Health Assembly has risen over time, and a large number of resolutions have been adopted, some in areas that are not high priorities for global health. To increase the strategic decisionmaking of WHO governing body meetings, WHO proposals include structuring debate around its priorities. WHO proposals for harmonizing the operations of its regional committees include aligning their meeting agendas and connecting their work more closely with that of the Executive Board. WHO also plans to strengthen the oversight role of its committee that reviews program, budget, and administrative issues.

Although WHO aims to strengthen its engagement with the many stakeholders directly involved in the global health sector and to improve the coherence of their efforts, it lacks a current proposal on how to achieve these aims. WHO's constitution describes two of its functions as (1) acting as the directing and coordinating authority on international health work and (2) establishing and maintaining effective collaboration with the UN, specialized agencies, and other global health organizations. Given the growing number of institutions—including foundations, partnerships, civil society organizations, and the private sector—that have a role in influencing global health policy, WHO reports that it is trying to determine how it can engage with a wide range of stakeholders. According to WHO, at the same time, it does not want to undermine its intergovernmental nature or open itself to undue influence by parties with vested interests.

In 2011, WHO proposed a forum to explore ways in which the major actors in global health could work more effectively together; however, WHO stakeholders did not support this proposal. WHO's concept paper proposed the idea of a "World Health Forum," an informal, multi-stakeholder body composed of representatives of governments, civil society organizations, private sector entities, and other relevant stakeholders. However, according to WHO, feedback from member states on this proposal was generally unsupportive because they did not want to create a forum that could potentially impinge upon the intergovernmental nature of WHO. In addition, some nongovernmental organizations were concerned that the proposed forum would allow private sector interests to influence decision-making in WHO. However, pharmaceutical industry representatives stated that the private sector has an important role to play in public health policy-making decisions. In May 2011, a group of nongovernmental organizations wrote a letter to WHO expressing concerns regarding the role of private bodies in the financing and governance of WHO. The nongovernmental organizations also expressed concern that the WHO reform proposals at the time did not adequately address the issue of how WHO planned to manage potential conflicts of interest for private institutions.

According to WHO, more discussion and consultation is necessary to identify how it will strengthen its engagement with external stakeholders. Since WHO set aside its World Health Forum proposal, WHO plans to consult with nongovernmental organizations on how it can effectively interact with them. In May 2012, member states requested that WHO present a draft policy document on its engagement with nongovernmental organizations to the Executive Board in January 2013. WHO also plans to hold a series of structured consultations concerning its relationship with private commercial entities and to develop a draft policy document on its guidelines for interacting with private entities to be presented to the Executive Board in May 2013.

WHO concerns in the area of global health governance also include a concern that, in light of the growing expansion of the number of global health initiatives and partnerships, a number of global health organizations have overlapping roles and responsibilities. For example, WHO recognizes a need to delineate the roles and responsibilities between itself; the Global Fund to Fight AIDS, Tuberculosis, and Malaria; and the GAVI Alliance, particularly in the area of providing technical assistance at the country level. WHO is involved in several formally structured partnerships, some hosted by WHO and others by independent entities that include WHO as part of their governing bodies. WHO reports that it aims to strengthen the Executive Board's oversight over its partnerships.

WHO Management Proposals and Actions Encompass a Wide Range of Areas

Management reforms encompass a broad range of areas, including efforts to (1) improve the predictability and flexibility of WHO's financing; (2) improve its human resource policies and practices; (3) strengthen WHO's results-based management, accountability, and transparency systems. According to WHO, the provision of stronger and more effective support to countries is a key outcome of its management reforms. At the November 2011 special session of the Executive Board, the Board approved WHO's management reform proposals in several areas and requested the development of proposals in other areas. To improve the predictability and flexibility of its financing, WHO proposed setting up a dialogue with donors after the approval of its program budget by the World Health Assembly, followed by a financing dialogue in which donors publicly make funding commitments that are aligned with the budget. To improve its human resource policies and practices, WHO proposed the development of a revised workforce model and contract types; streamlined recruitment and selection processes; improved performance management processes; a staff mobility and rotation framework; and enhanced staff development and learning opportunities. To strengthen WHO's accountability, and transparency systems, WHO proposed a strengthened internal control framework and conflict of interest policy; increased capacity of its audit and oversight office; improved monitoring and reporting; and the establishment of an information disclosure policy and an ethics office. WHO has begun implementing some of its management reform proposals. For example, according to WHO, it took steps to strengthen the staffing of its internal audit and oversight office and developed a draft formal evaluation policy for consideration and approval by the WHO Executive Board. According to WHO officials, although member states approved the implementation of many WHO management reform proposals, they requested that WHO further develop its proposals to increase the flexibility and transparency of WHO financing and present its proposals to the Executive Board in January 2013.

Multiple Challenges Could Impede the Successful Implementation of WHO Reform

Multiple challenges could affect the success of WHO reform implementation. WHO developed a high-level implementation and monitoring framework that included reform objectives, selected activities, 1-year and 3-year milestones, and intended results for consideration by the May 2012 World Health Assembly. For example, to improve WHO's human resources practices, WHO set a 1-year milestone of conducting regular reviews of its staffing levels and a 3-year milestone of comprehensively integrating its human resources planning into its program planning and budgeting processes. WHO's intended result for these efforts is staffing that is more closely matched to needs at all levels of the organization. We previously reported that, when undergoing an organizational change, it is important to establish implementation goals, a timeline, estimated costs for achieving the goals, and performance measures—all of which help build momentum and monitor progress.[16] While the framework contains some of these elements, WHO has not yet identified the estimated costs for the implementation of its reform program or defined performance measures, which would serve as an objective means by which to track the organization's progress in achieving its reform objectives. WHO officials have noted that they are currently developing an implementation plan that will include input from its member states and regional and country offices. Officials also noted that the components of its reform agenda will be implemented at various stages, and that as its reform efforts proceed, WHO will provide periodic updates on its progress to its governing bodies. Key challenges that could impede WHO's ability to successfully implement its reform proposals include the following:

- *Availability of sufficient resources.* According to WHO officials, implementation of its reform proposals will require financial and technical resources, and some of its reform proposals have significant resource implications, which must be carefully considered.[17]

- *Extent of support from internal and external WHO stakeholders.* Changes to WHO's established structures and processes will require support and commitment from WHO's internal and external stakeholders. Stakeholders raised concerns that, due to the autonomous nature of WHO's regional offices, WHO's reform proposals might not be implemented uniformly across the entire organization. In addition, WHO proposals to increase delegation of authority and strengthen its country offices will require the support of WHO's regional governing bodies and offices. WHO will require the support and consensus of member states to carry its reform proposals forward.

---

[16]GAO-03-669.

[17]WHO's budget for the development phase of the reform is about $6.27 million and includes costs for consultations and meetings of the governing bodies, secretariat costs, and the independent evaluation. According to WHO, member states have provided about $3.04 million in funding thus far, resulting in a funding gap of about $3.23 million.

The United States Has Provided Input into WHO's Reform Agenda, Particularly in Transparency and Accountability Proposals, but State's Tool for Monitoring Progress Could be Enhanced

The United States has provided input into WHO's reform agenda, particularly in the areas of transparency and accountability, but State's tool to assess the progress of management reforms could be enhanced. On priority-setting, the United States has advocated for WHO to maintain its focus on certain functions such as setting norms and standards for international health. On consultations on governance, the U.S. delegation has commented on a range of proposals put forth by WHO, including those on engagement with other global health stakeholders. On management reforms, the United States has supported increased transparency and accountability mechanisms at WHO; however, State's tool for monitoring progress in this area could be enhanced.

The United States Has Provided Input on WHO Consultations on Priority-Setting and Governance

Priority-setting

The United States has advocated for WHO to maintain its focus on setting standards and guidelines, as well as other global health goals.

In priority-setting consultations, the U.S. delegation has advocated for WHO to maintain its focus on normative functions such as setting standards and guidelines, as well as other areas such as health security and communicable diseases. According to talking points used in preparation for governing body meetings, the U.S. delegation has stressed the need for WHO to remain focused on its core functions of setting standards and guidelines for global health. HHS officials noted that one of the main challenges facing WHO is the development of a narrower set of clear priorities and the need to focus on areas where it has a strategic advantage. According to State and HHS officials, the United States advocated that WHO maintain its focus on normative-setting functions such as setting norms and standards for international health. HHS officials stated that WHO is uniquely positioned to be the international authoritative body for establishing rules and technical standards and conducting monitoring activities. For example, WHO is the major international counterpart for CDC on outbreak control and identifying potential global health threats. Officials from State and USUN-Geneva also stated that U.S. priorities for WHO are focused on its normative functions of setting standards and guidelines. For example, State officials noted that the U.S. government wants WHO to focus on its processes to ensure safe medicines and vaccines, including WHO's drug prequalification process and essential medicines list. These U.S. officials stated that WHO's main mission should be to remain the international authority for global health on norms and standards.

The U.S. delegation also advocated for a number of other health priorities for WHO, including improving health security and preventing communicable diseases. According to talking points used in preparation for governing body meetings, the U.S. delegation highlighted the importance of including health security and communicable diseases among WHO's priorities. In addition, State and USUN-Geneva officials cited health security as a key U.S. priority for WHO. State officials noted that U.S. priorities for global health involve protecting the health of Americans at home and abroad; the health security functions of WHO are thus important for achieving this goal. An official from USUN-Geneva noted that health security involves a number of components such as enhancing pandemic preparedness, setting international health norms, and eradicating certain diseases such as small pox, and that WHO is in a unique position to provide leadership in these areas. HHS and State officials also stated that WHO is a critical partner with the United States in fighting communicable diseases such as polio and influenza. A State budget document stated that the U.S. benefits from WHO-sponsored cooperation on vital aspects of global health security, including containing the HIV/AIDS pandemic, preventing the spread of avian influenza and other emerging diseases, and addressing long-term threats to health such as bioterrorism and the spread of chronic diseases.

Governance

The United States has provided input on WHO proposals.

The United States has provided input on a range of WHO proposals in the governance area, according to a U.S. government document used in preparation for governing body meetings. For example, the U.S. delegation supported WHO proposals to improve engagement between WHO and outside stakeholders, such as other global health organizations. In addition, the United States commented on WHO proposals related to the frequency of governing body meetings and the linkages between regional and global policies and strategies. Specifically, the United States favors having the regions adapt global policies and strategies, rather than repeating the process of policy and strategy development at the regional level. In governance consultations, the U.S. delegation also pushed for a greater effort to define WHO's strategic engagement in partnerships and the degree to which the partnerships meet WHO's interests.

The United States Has Supported a Management Reform Agenda for Greater Transparency and Accountability, but State's Tool to Assess Progress in These Areas Could be Enhanced

Management Reforms

The United States has supported increased transparency and accountability and improvements to budgeting and planning at WHO.

The United States has supported an agenda for greater transparency and accountability for WHO management reforms. According to State officials, State's Bureau of International Organization Affairs takes the lead for the U.S. government on issues related to management reform and is responsible for pursuing management reforms throughout the UN system, including WHO. U.S. officials mentioned a number of U.S. goals in this area, including improving internal and external oversight mechanisms, budgeting and planning processes, and human resources and administrative reforms. According to State officials, cost effectiveness, efficiency, accountability, and monitoring and evaluation are key U.S. priorities for WHO reform.

The U.S. delegation has taken steps to advocate for a number of reforms to improve WHO's internal and external oversight mechanisms. According to State officials, the United States encouraged the reestablishment of an independent audit committee for WHO. The previous audit committee was disbanded in 2005 amid concerns about its effectiveness, and a revamped audit committee was established in 2009. Officials also noted that State supports WHO in establishing a dedicated ethics office, which is currently under consideration as part of the proposed reforms. For example, according to WHO officials, the U.S. delegation introduced a proposal that would require the newly formed ethics office to report directly to the Program Budget and Administration Committee, thereby enhancing the independence of the office. In addition, according to a USUN-Geneva official, the United States pushed for improved independent evaluation at WHO, and WHO agreed in November 2011 to conduct an independent evaluation as an input into the reform process.

According to officials from USUN-Geneva, two additional management-related goals for the United States include improvements in the budgeting and planning process and human resources and administrative reforms. Specifically, the United States has emphasized that WHO makes the necessary changes to its budgeting and planning system to ensure that WHO resources are aligned with its stated objectives. For example, according to WHO officials, the U.S. delegation offered an amendment at the May 2012 Executive Board meeting to hold a special meeting of the Program Budget and Administration Committee in late 2012 in order to discuss WHO financing as well as other reform issues. The U.S. delegation also has advocated for human resources and personnel reforms to ensure that WHO staff have the appropriate skill set for the organization's current needs. In particular, according to talking points prepared for governing body meetings, the United States pushed for a new workforce model to distinguish long-term functions from time-limited projects and for a skills profile of staff at each level of the organization as a way to improve the organization's effectiveness and flexibility. Officials from USUN-Geneva have met with officials from the WHO human resource office to advocate for reforms in this area. The United States also advocated to harmonize recruitment policies, increase the speed of hiring, improve performance management processes, and enhance staff development and learning. USUN-Geneva officials noted that WHO is taking steps to respond to the concerns and proposals raised by the United States and other member states as part of the reform agenda.

Management Reforms

State has developed a tool for monitoring progress in transparency and accountability, but lacks sufficient guidance on completing assessments.

State established an assessment tool to measure progress on transparency and accountability mechanisms, a tool that could assist in monitoring the progress of management reforms. State's UNTAI tool is used to assess approximately 20 UN agencies, including WHO, to monitor progress on eight goals related to transparency and accountability, with a number of specific benchmarks in each category. For example, the UNTAI goal "effective oversight arrangements" contains six benchmarks, including whether the external audit reports are publicly available online and if there are term limits for the external auditor. According to State officials, the UNTAI tool is not intended to cover the full range of U.S. goals and priorities in the area of management reform. For instance, the assessment tool does not cover certain U.S. priorities such as human resources and personnel systems, which is another key component of management reform.

UNTAI is a useful tool for guiding U.S. priorities and engagement on certain management issues. According to State officials, State assigned WHO "above average" scores on UNTAI criteria relative to other UN organizations, and the assessment identified certain areas for improvement. State's UNTAI assessment scored WHO well in areas related to whistleblower protection and conflicts-of-interest policies. However, the WHO UNTAI assessment identified areas for improvement in certain areas, such as maintaining an independent ethics function. According to State officials, as a result of the goals laid out in UNTAI, the U.S. delegation pushed for the establishment of an independent audit committee at WHO. A USUN-Geneva official noted that the UNTAI assessment is used to guide U.S. priorities and engagement on issues related to transparency and accountability and to sharpen the U.S. position in these areas.

To conduct the UNTAI assessment, officials can use a number of strategies, according to State officials. State officials at the mission carry out the assessments, either by completing the tool themselves, or providing it to the UN organization to complete. For example, State officials at the mission can collect information to complete the assessment by interviewing officials from the UN agency, such as representatives of an ethics or management office. In some cases, the UNTAI assessment tool is provided to UN agency representatives as a self-assessment exercise. According to State officials, the mission vets the completed assessments and sends them to Washington for review. For example, the most recent UNTAI assessment for WHO, covering fiscal year 2011, was completed by WHO representatives and verified by officials from USUN-Geneva and State in Washington, D.C.

According to State officials, State has provided some general guidelines for completing UNTAI assessments to State officials at the mission in addition to providing technical and agency-specific advice on an as-needed basis. State provided information on the UNTAI goals and benchmarks through cables to officials in the field in 2008 and 2011. State officials noted that questions about the assessment tool are answered through correspondence between the missions and State in Washington. In addition, some State officials at the mission choose to provide additional information with the assessment; however, State does not require that supporting documentation accompany the assessments. State officials at the mission completing the assessments are asked to defend the assigned ratings to State officials in Washington and make an evidence-based case for the assigned scores. According to State officials, State consulted with officials in the field to develop the assessment tool and such a consultative process helped to facilitate a shared understanding among those completing and reviewing the assessments. State officials also noted that the process of reviewing the UNTAI reports in Washington helps to minimize errors, omissions, and inconsistencies, but that this process does not fully mitigate risks to data reliability. State officials mentioned that they are considering distributing a list of frequently asked questions to officers in the field to aid in completing the assessment in the upcoming fiscal year. In addition, State officials we spoke with stated that the UNTAI tool was updated for 2011 and that they recognize that areas for improvement and clarification may still exist, as they often do with surveys and data collection instruments. An official at USUN-Geneva welcomed improved guidance noting that this would assist officials in the field in completing the assessment tool.

We found some weaknesses in State's UNTAI assessment of WHO, including an ambiguous rationale for State's scores on certain benchmarks. In reviewing State's WHO UNTAI assessment, we could not find support for State's scoring on 14 of 50 benchmarks. For example, we could not find support for State's determination that WHO's evaluation and management functions are autonomous. The comments submitted with the UNTAI assessment stated that most evaluation is decentralized and commissioned under individual technical areas. Therefore, the evaluation function is not functionally separate at an organizational level from those responsible for the design and implementation of the programs and operations evaluated, as specified in the UNTAI benchmarks. In addition, State's WHO UNTAI assessment concluded that WHO consistently and objectively applied its policy on program support costs, which was approved by the member states; however, this policy does not appear to be consistently applied. The program support cost policy requires that 13 percent of all voluntary funding contributions are allocated to reimburse WHO for administering projects of voluntarily funded programs. However, according to WHO officials, many donors negotiate a program support charge averaging around 7 percent, rather than the standard rate of 13 percent, for their voluntary contributions.

We also found that State's definitions of certain benchmarks used in State's UNTAI tool were unclear and may lead to data reliability concerns. We analyzed State's UNTAI tool to assess whether the tool is likely to gather accurate and consistent data. We found that 15 of 50 benchmarks in the UNTAI assessment tool required the judgment of the reviewer, due to the subject matter expertise required to complete the assessment, the lack of clarity on the benchmark definitions, or both. Certain benchmarks require an understanding of specific subject areas to accurately determine whether the benchmark has been met, and not all State officials completing the assessments have the required expertise in each area to make an accurate judgment. For example, the benchmark indicating whether or not the organization has an independent, transparent, effective, and fair bid protest process requires some knowledge related to acquisition and procurement rules to make such a determination. In addition, certain benchmarks use ambiguous or indefinite terminology, requiring the assessor to define the meaning of the terms before they can assess whether the benchmark has been met. For example, the determination of whether the organization has adequate staff and financial resources allocated to the evaluation function requires some judgment about the definition of adequate in this context. The UNTAI tool does not provide sufficient guidance to reviewers to assist in making these judgments and does not require documentation from the assessor to explain how such a judgment was made. See appendix II for further information on GAO's analysis of the benchmarks in State's UNTAI assessment tool.

Conclusions

WHO has undertaken an ambitious and comprehensive agenda for reform; however, as with other organizations undergoing major transformational change such as broad reforms, WHO faces potential challenges throughout implementation. WHO's high-level implementation and monitoring framework includes important elements for planning organizational change, such as reform objectives, 1-year and 3-year milestones, and intended results. In addition, WHO is currently developing a detailed implementation plan, which would help WHO achieve its goals, including the creation of performance indicators to measure progress and identification of the estimated costs for implementing its broad reform agenda. Thus, success of WHO reform depends on the ability of WHO to sustain its efforts to establish such a comprehensive reform implementation plan, as well as other essential elements including consensus from member states and other internal and external stakeholders. The U.S. delegation has participated in numerous consultations on WHO reform and has been supportive of reforms to improve the efficiency and effectiveness of the organization. The United States has been particularly supportive of WHO's focus on its core functions of setting standards and guidelines, as well as a set of reforms improving the transparency and accountability mechanisms of the organization. State's UNTAI assessment is a useful tool for shaping U.S. engagement with WHO and monitoring WHO progress in implementing certain management reforms related to UNTAI goals and benchmarks. However, there are weaknesses in the UNTAI assessment tool that generate concerns over the reliability of the information generated in these assessments, including the ambiguous rationale for State's scores in particular areas and the lack of clarity in the definitions of certain benchmarks. Therefore, ensuring that the performance information resulting from the UNTAI assessment is useful and accurate is crucial for State's ability to continue advocating for improvements at WHO and monitor WHO reform implementation in certain areas of management reform.

Recommendation for Executive Action

To improve U.S. assessment of WHO reform, we recommend that the Secretary of State enhance its guidance on completing State's assessment tool for monitoring WHO's progress in implementing transparency and accountability reforms by including, for example, a requirement to collect and submit supporting documentation with completed assessments.

Agency Comments and Our Evaluation

We requested comments on a draft of this report from the Departments of State and HHS, USAID, and WHO. State and WHO provided written comments that are reprinted in appendixes III and IV of this report. HHS and USAID did not provide written comments on this report.

State generally endorsed the main findings and conclusions of our report and concurred that WHO has undertaken an ambitious and comprehensive agenda for reform. State also agreed that the United States has advocated for and provided input into WHO's reform agenda, particularly in the areas of management, budgeting and planning, priority setting, governance, and financing. State agreed that its process for conducting its UNTAI assessment could be strengthened and accepted our recommendation to revise its guidance for completing these assessments. State noted that it is in the process of updating its assessment tool and plans to issue expanded guidance prior to the fiscal year 2012 ratings. State also clarified the context regarding its assessments. State noted that we overstated the need for subject matter expertise in determining whether some benchmarks on the UNTAI assessment tool have been met. We recognize that some officers in the field completing the assessment may benefit from the expertise of those in the Bureau of International Organization Affairs. However, we maintain that the UNTAI tool does not provide sufficient guidance to reviewers to assist in making these judgments and that this could lead to potential data reliability concerns. Furthermore, according to an official at USUN-Geneva, improved guidance would be welcome and would help officials in the field complete the assessment tool. In addition, State mentioned the need to balance the requirement for supporting documentation with the need to minimize the reporting burden on missions, WHO, and other UN organizations. We recognize State's concern about overburdening missions with reporting requirements and maintain that revised guidance would benefit both the missions and officers in Washington in preparing and reviewing these assessments.

In its comments, WHO concurred with the main conclusions of our report and stated that our review provides an important framework against which WHO and its member states can evaluate the reform's direction. WHO agreed that the reform proposals respond to the challenges identified by stakeholders, and that the consultation process has been inclusive and transparent. In addition, WHO noted that our conclusions broadly converge with those of the evaluation conducted by WHO's External Auditor. WHO also recognized that the development of a detailed implementation plan will be critical to ensure successful institutional change.

State, HHS, USAID, and WHO also provided technical comments that we have incorporated into this report, as appropriate.

As agreed with your offices, unless you publicly announce the contents of this report earlier, we plan no further distribution until 30 days from the report date. At that time, we will send copies to interested congressional committees, the Secretaries of State and HHS, the Administrator of USAID, the U.S. Permanent Representative to the UN in Geneva, the Director-General of WHO, and other interested parties. In addition, the report will be available at no charge on the GAO website at http://www.gao.gov.

If you or your staff have any questions about this report, please contact me at (202) 512-9601 or melitot@gao.gov. Contact points for our Offices of Congressional Relations and Public Affairs may be found on the last page of this report. GAO staff who made major contributions to this report are listed in appendix V.

Sincerely yours,
Thomas Melito
Director, International Affairs and Trade

Appendix I: Scope and Methodology

This report examines (1) the steps the World Health Organization (WHO) has taken to develop and implement a reform agenda that aligns with the challenges identified by the organization, its member states, and other stakeholders; and (2) the input the United States has provided to WHO reforms.

To assess the steps that WHO has taken to develop and implement a reform agenda that aligns with the challenges identified by the organization, its member states, and other stakeholders, we conducted interviews in Washington, D.C., and in Geneva, Switzerland, with WHO officials, representatives of member states to the WHO, and a range of WHO stakeholders. We obtained their views on the challenges WHO faces and whether these challenges align with those addressed in WHO's reform agenda. We also solicited their views on the steps WHO has taken to consult with internal and external stakeholders in developing and implementing its reform agenda. We interviewed WHO officials based in its headquarters office, six regional offices, and five country offices, including representatives of WHO's reform team, task force on reform, and headquarters staff association. We interviewed officials from the U.S. Departments of State (State), Health and Human Services (HHS), Centers for Disease Control and Prevention (CDC), U.S. Agency for International Development (USAID), and officials representing 15 other member states to WHO. We interviewed representatives from institutions such as the Global Fund to Fight AIDS, Tuberculosis, and Malaria and the GAVI Alliance;[1] nongovernmental organizations, such as Doctors without Borders and the Institute of Medicine; and the Bill & Melinda Gates Foundation, one of the largest donors to the WHO. We also met with representatives of UN agencies, such as UNAIDS and the United Nations Development Program; private sector entities, including U.S. and international pharmaceutical research associations; and two research centers that review global health issues. In addition, we reviewed WHO documents on its reform agenda and process, including its evaluation plans and its implementation and monitoring framework for reform.

To examine U.S. support for WHO reforms, we met with officials from State, HHS, CDC, and USAID. We also conducted field work in Geneva, Switzerland, to meet with officials from USUN-Geneva, WHO, and other

---

[1]The GAVI Alliance was formerly known as the Global Alliance for Vaccines and Immunization.

member state missions to learn about U.S. participation in WHO reform discussions and collaboration with other WHO member states. We collected and reviewed relevant U.S. government documents, including budget documents, strategies, position papers, talking points, and speeches. Based on interviews with U.S. government officials and U.S. government documents, we conducted an analysis to identify possible U.S. government priorities for WHO reform. We also collected and analyzed data from State, HHS, CDC, and USAID on U.S. funding contributions to WHO. We determined that these data were sufficiently reliable for the purposes of presenting specific agency contributions to WHO.

To examine State's United Nations Transparency and Accountability Initiative (UNTAI) tool to measure the performance and progress of UN agencies, including WHO, on transparency and accountability, we interviewed State officials at State's Bureau of International Organization Affairs, which developed and uses the assessment tool. To examine the results of State's assessment of WHO using the UNTAI tool, we interviewed officials at USUN-Geneva who are involved in completing the assessment of WHO. We also systematically reviewed State's WHO UNTAI report to verify the basis for State's determinations on each benchmark. Specifically, we examined State's assigned score for each benchmark against the information WHO provided, noting benchmarks where the support for State's determination was not clear. In addition, we reviewed the specific benchmarks used in State's UNTAI tool to determine potential threats to the accuracy and consistency of the resulting assessments. To do so, we developed definitions of the types of judgment necessary to implement the tools, and two analysts independently applied those definitions to each benchmark. They then met to compare and resolve any differences. The two analysts agreed upon resolutions until there was 100 percent agreement on the coding. Finally, we met with officials from State's Bureau of International Organization Affairs about the results of our review of the benchmarks and our analysis of WHO's assessment results.

We conducted this performance audit from August 2011 to July 2012 in accordance with generally accepted government auditing standards. Those standards require that we plan and perform the audit to obtain sufficient, appropriate evidence to provide a reasonable basis for our findings and conclusions based on our audit objectives. We believe the evidence obtained provides a reasonable basis for our findings and conclusions based on our audit objectives.

Appendix II: GAO Assessment of State's UNTAI Assessment Tool

We performed a review of State's United Nations Transparency and Accountability Initiative (UNTAI) assessment tool to better understand its potential usefulness for supporting State's monitoring of management reforms. The usefulness of the data collected by the tool is affected by the degree to which the resulting data are complete and accurate,[1] which requires that the data gathered are clear and well defined enough to attain consistent results.[2] We reviewed the specific benchmarks used in State's UNTAI tool to determine potential risks to the accuracy and consistency of the resulting assessments.[3]

GAO's Assessment Methodology

In conducting our analysis, we developed a methodology for determining if the benchmarks in the assessment were clear and sufficiently defined to yield similar results when applied by different individuals. We found that the largest area of concern resulted from the judgment required when evaluating benchmarks. (A full description of our coding methodology and analysis can be found in app. I).

We identified the following two types of judgment necessary to implement the tool for 15 UNTAI benchmarks:

1. *Subject matter expertise* - Benchmarks that require an understanding of a specific area of knowledge to make an accurate determination. These are benchmarks for which professional judgment is necessary to accurately determine if the benchmark has been met. For example, one benchmark related to the training and qualification of procurement officials would require subject matter expertise in procurement to understand what qualifications or training might be appropriate for procurement professionals.

---

[1]*Government Performance: GPRA Modernization Act Provides Opportunities to Help Address Fiscal, Performance, and Management Challenges*, GAO-11-466T (Washington, D.C.: Mar. 16, 2011).

[2]*Auditing and Financial Management: Assessing the Reliability of Computer-Processed Data*, GAO-09-680G (Washington, D.C.: Jul. 1, 2009).

[3]Other factors relating to usefulness of information include completeness, timeliness, and ease of use. We limit the focus to accuracy and consistency because UNTAI is not the only tool State uses to monitor management reforms, and because determining whether the information produced using UNTAI is complete, timely, or easily used depends on the information State may obtain through other methods.

2. *Definitional judgment* - Benchmarks that require a determination of scope, size, or meaning. These are benchmarks in which ambiguous terminology or imprecise terms are used, which the assessor must define to assess whether the benchmark has been met. For example, this benchmark would require definitional judgment to determine if the level of qualifications and training would make an individual "qualified and trained." Definitional judgment would also be needed to determine the proportion of the total number of professionals who must be "qualified and trained" for the agency to meet that benchmark.

Judgment Is Needed for 15 of 50 Benchmarks in State's Assessment Tool

We determined that 35 of the 50 benchmarks in UNTAI (70 percent) require neither subject matter expertise nor definitional judgment. Of the remaining 15 benchmarks, 5 (10 percent) require both definitional judgment and subject matter expertise to be assessed, 4 (8 percent) require subject matter expertise, and 6 (12 percent) require definitional judgment, which may affect the accuracy and consistency of the results for those benchmarks.

Of the nine benchmarks where subject matter expertise was required, we found knowledge would be needed in five relevant areas to complete the assessment: training and development, acquisitions and procurement, UN policies and practices, auditing and evaluation, and accounting standards. The accuracy and consistency of the individual determinations will depend, in part, on the assessors' expertise in these five areas, and on their definitional judgment relative to other assessors. For example, one benchmark asks whether "funding arrangements facilitate effective and independent evaluations of the organization's activities." This benchmark requires subject matter expertise related to auditing and evaluation and definitional judgment about effectiveness to accurately assess the relevant UN agency. This judgment creates the potential that two assessors with different levels of subject matter expertise and who apply different definitional judgments could rate the same program differently. The potential variation in judgment and knowledge of the assessor could make the overall score of the UN agency vary from 2 to 5 points on UNTAI's 5-point scale. Guidance on how to assess each of these benchmarks would serve to mitigate the need for judgment and reduce the risk of inconsistency in the assessments.

Appendix III: Comments from the Department of State

Note: GAO comments supplementing those in the report text appear at the end of this appendix.

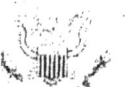

United States Department of State
Comptroller
1969 Dyess Drive
Charleston, SC 29405

JUL 0 9 2012

Dr. Loren Yager
Managing Director
International Affairs and Trade
Government Accountability Office
441 G Street, N.W.
Washington, D.C. 20548-0001

Dear Dr. Yager:

We appreciate the opportunity to review your draft report, "WORLD HEALTH ORGANIZATION: Reform Agenda Developed, but U.S. Actions to Monitor Progress Could be Enhanced" GAO Job Code 320862.

The enclosed Department of State comments are provided for incorporation with this letter as an appendix to the final report.

If you have any questions concerning this response, please contact Matt Glockner, Program Analyst, Bureau of International Organization Affairs at (202) 647-6413.

Sincerely,

James L. Millette

cc: GAO – Thomas Melito
       IO – Esther D. Brimmer
       State/OIG – Evelyn Klemstine

Department of State Comments on GAO Draft Report

**WORLD HEALTH ORGANIZATION: Reform Agenda Developed, but U.S.
Actions to Monitor Progress Could be Enhanced
(GAO-12-722, GAO Code 320862)**

Thank you for the opportunity to comment on your draft report entitled
*WORLD HEALTH ORGANIZATION: Reform Agenda Developed. but U.S.
Actions to Monitor Progress Could be Enhanced.* The Department of State has
long been an ardent supporter of reform at the World Health Organization (WHO)
and throughout the wider UN system and has, in particular, strongly supported the
WHO reform agenda that started in earnest in 2010. The GAO's report provides
timely and useful information on a number of aspects of the WHO reform agenda.

The Department of State generally endorses the main findings and
conclusions contained in the GAO report. We are pleased that the GAO report
found that the United States has advocated for and provided input into WHO's
reform agenda, particularly in the areas of management and improvements to
budgeting and planning, as well as priority setting, governance, and financing, and
that the United States established a useful assessment tool to measure progress on
specific reforms. We are also pleased the report acknowledges that WHO has
undertaken and continues with an ambitious and comprehensive agenda for
reforms focused on priority-setting, governance, and management reforms and has
done so in a consultative manner with its Member States and stakeholders. We
particularly value that the report notes that the long-term success of WHO reform
depends on the ability of WHO to sustain its efforts through a comprehensive
implementation plan, and a consensus from internal and external stakeholders.

The report makes one recommendation, relating to guidance for utilizing the
Department's assessment tool for monitoring progress via the U.S.-sponsored
United Nations Transparency and Accountability Initiative (UNTAI). We agree
that the UNTAI assessment process could be strengthened and accept GAO's
recommendation to revise guidance for completing the annual assessment tool.
The Department of State is in the process of updating the assessment tool and plans
to issue expanded guidance prior to the FY 2012 rating. The Department of State
would also like to make some clarifications and amplifications concerning UNTAI.

First, we would like to emphasize that although GAO's recommendation
may be directed toward the use of the assessment tool for WHO, UNTAI is an
effort that involves 24 organizations in the UN system including WHO, and as

2

such the recommendation has implications that extend beyond the scope of the present GAO report on WHO. We appreciate GAO's observations related to WHO's assessment and are studying how these might be applied to the broader UNTAI project.

Second, the assessment tool is not designed to be an audit or systematic evaluation of WHO management reforms or those of any other UN organization. The annual assessment is a limited scope survey of where WHO and other UN organizations stand on various management reform goals. While we appreciate the observations generated by the involvement of GAO's methodologist, we developed UNTAI as a broad assessment tool to identify weaknesses and prioritize our engagement on reforms at WHO and elsewhere. We appreciate GAO's acknowledgement that UNTAI has helped achieve management reforms at WHO such as the establishment of an audit committee. We believe that the assessment process will continue to encourage WHO to make progress on accountability and transparency reforms.

See comment 1.

Third, we believe that GAO has overstated the need for subject matter expertise in determining whether some benchmarks on the UNTAI assessment tool have been met. The Office of Management Policy and Resources in the Bureau of International Organization Affairs designed the UNTAI assessment tool in consultation with Missions and other relevant offices and bureaus within the Department. The Office regularly answers subject matter and agency specific questions on the assessments for WHO and other UN organizations. In addition, the Office carefully reviews UNTAI reports to help minimize errors, omissions, and inconsistencies. We are in the process of developing a list of Frequently Asked Questions that will be posted on the Department's intranet site for use by Missions. We believe that the existing review process combined with planned revisions and enhancements to the guidance for completing the assessment tool will address GAO's concerns.

See comment 2.

Finally, the Department would like to stress that it must balance a requirement for supporting documentation with the need to minimize the burden on Missions, the WHO, and other UN organizations. The UNTAI reporting process as it currently stands involves a significant investment of staff time by Missions and officers in Washington to prepare and review annual assessments. Collection and submission of supporting documentation could be beneficial and will be encouraged across the board; however, we will not specifically require such documentation except for instances where we might have specific questions or concerns about a particular benchmark or rating. The GAO report cites examples

3

where such follow-up would be useful to better enable the Department to monitor the status of WHO reforms and advocate for further progress.

As the report illustrates, WHO has developed a reform agenda that is generally aligned with the priorities of its stakeholders. WHO has been taking positive steps to implement reforms in the areas of priority-setting, governance, and management. We appreciate the report's acknowledgment that the United States has been actively involved in shaping and advancing the reform agenda, and particularly our vigorous engagement on improving WHO's transparency and accountability mechanisms. We remain committed to working with WHO and other member states to make further progress on the full range of reforms.

The following are GAO's comments on the Department of State's letter dated July 9, 2012.

GAO Comments

1. We recognize that some officers in the field completing the assessment may benefit from the expertise of those in the Bureau of International Organization Affairs. However, we maintain that the UNTAI tool does not provide sufficient guidance to reviewers to assist in making these judgments and that this could lead to potential data reliability concerns. Furthermore, according to an official at USUN-Geneva, improved guidance would be welcome and would help officials in the field complete the assessment tool.

2. We recognize State's concern about overburdening missions with reporting requirements and maintain that revised guidance would benefit both the missions and officers in Washington in preparing and reviewing these assessments.

Appendix IV: Comments from the World Health Organization

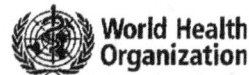

World Health Organization

20, AVENUE APPIA – CH-1211 GENEVA 27 – SWITZERLAND – TEL CENTRAL +41 22 791 2111 – FAX CENTRAL +41 22 791 3111 – WWW.WHO.INT

Tel. direct: +41 22 791
Fax direct: +41 22 791
E-mail :

In reply please
refer to:

Your reference:

Mr Thomas Melito
Director, International Affairs and Trade
U.S. Government Accountability
Office
441 G Street, N.W.
Washington, D.C. 20548

3 July 2012

Dear Mr Melito,

***Response to the United States Government Accountability Report entitled,
"World Health Organization: Reform Agenda Developed, but U.S. Actions to
Monitor Progress Could be Enhanced" by the World Health Organization***

The World Health Organization (WHO) welcomes the report issued by the United States Government Accountability Office (GAO) entitled *"World Health Organization – Reform Agenda Developed, but U.S. Actions to Monitor Progress Could be Enhanced."* WHO appreciates the opportunity to provide feedback on the report and the United States Government's strong interest in the reform of WHO. WHO acknowledges that GAO's performance audit included a detailed review of reform-related documentation and consultations with Member States and a range of global health stakeholders. WHO shares the U.S. Government's interest in seeing WHO improve performance and organizational efficiency underpinned by principles of accountability and transparency.

The detailed examination undertaken by GAO provides an important framework against which WHO and its Member States can evaluate the direction of the programme of reform in the context of current challenges facing the Organization. In this regard, WHO particularly welcomes GAO's primary conclusions that the proposals which comprise WHO's reform agenda respond to the challenges identified by stakeholders, and that the process of consultation has been inclusive and transparent. WHO notes that these conclusions broadly converge with those of the evaluation conducted by WHO's External Auditor. In particular both studies stress the importance of improving the predictability and flexibility of the Organization's financing, and of programmatic reforms that will ensure clear priority-setting.

منظمة الصحة العالمية · 世界卫生组织
Organisation mondiale de la Santé · Всемирная организация здравоохранения · Organización Mundial de la Salud

Page 2

As the process of reform moves from development to implementation, WHO is focusing on the multiple challenges that might impede progress. Two of the specific challenges observed in the GAO report – namely the availability of sufficient resources, and the extent of support from internal and external WHO stakeholders – are equally of concern to WHO. In this regard, WHO is proceeding with measures designed to address the funding of reform, and, continuing extensive, internal and external consultative processes aiming to guide Organizational changes. Specifically, as noted in the GAO report, WHO recognizes that the development of a detailed implementation plan outlining goals, milestones, costs and indicators to monitor and measure the success of implementation, will be critical to ensure successful, institutional change. WHO welcomes the analysis that the study provides and notes that the key U.S. priorities   cost effectiveness, efficiency, accountability and monitoring and evaluation – underscore and reflect the primary objectives of WHO's programme of reform.

Yours Sincerely,

Dr Margaret Chan
Director-General

منظمة الصحة العالمية • 世界卫生组织
Organisation mondiale de la Santé • Всемирная организация здравоохранения • Organización Mundial de la Salud

Appendix V: GAO Contact and Staff Acknowledgments

GAO Contact	Thomas Melito, (202) 512-9601, or melitot@gao.gov
Staff Acknowledgments	In addition to the contact named above, Joy Labez (Assistant Director), Diana Blumenfeld, Debbie Chung, Lynn Cothern, Karen Deans, Mark Dowling, Etana Finkler, Emily Gupta, Steven Putansu, Jena Sinkfield, R.G. Steinman, Teresa Tucker, and Sarah Veale made key contributions to this report. Gifford Howland and Kara Marshall provided additional technical assistance.

Related GAO Products

United Nations: Improved Reporting and Member States' Consensus Needed for Food and Agriculture Organization's Reform Plan. GAO-11-922. Washington, D.C.: September 29, 2011.

UN Internal Oversight: Progress Made on Independence and Staffing Issues, but Further Actions Are Needed. GAO-11-871. Washington, D.C.: September 20, 2011.

United Nations: Management Reforms and Operational Issues. GAO-08-246T. Washington, D.C.: January 24, 2008.

United Nations: Progress on Management Reform Efforts Has Varied. GAO-08-84. Washington, D.C.: November 14, 2007.

United Nations Organizations: Oversight and Accountability Could Be Strengthened by Further Instituting International Best Practices. GAO-07-597. Washington, D.C.: June 18, 2007.

United Nations: Management Reforms Progressing Slowly with Many Awaiting General Assembly Review. GAO-07-14. Washington, D.C.: October 5, 2006.

United Nations: Weaknesses in Internal Oversight and Procurement Could Affect the Effective Implementation of the Planned Renovation. GAO-06-877T. Washington, D.C.: June 20, 2006.

United Nations: Oil for Food Program Provides Lessons for Future Sanctions and Ongoing Reform. GAO-06-711T. Washington, D.C.: May 2, 2006.

United Nations: Internal Oversight and Procurement Controls and Processes Need Strengthening. GAO-06-710T. Washington, D.C.: April 27, 2006.

United Nations: Funding Arrangements Impede Independence of Internal Auditors. GAO-06-575. Washington, D.C.: April 25, 2006.

United Nations: Lessons Learned from Oil for Food Program Indicate the Need to Strengthen UN Internal Controls and Oversight. GAO-06-330. Washington, D.C.: April 25, 2006.

United Nations: Procurement Internal Controls Are Weak. GAO-06-577. Washington, D.C.: April 25, 2006.

United Nations: Preliminary Observations on Internal Oversight and Procurement Practices. GAO-06-226T. Washington, D.C.: October 31, 2005.

United Nations: Sustained Oversight Is Needed for Reforms to Achieve Lasting Results. GAO-05-392T. Washington, D.C.: March 2, 2005.

United Nations: Reforms Progressing, but Comprehensive Assessments Needed to Measure Impact. GAO-04-339. Washington, D.C.; February 13, 2004.

United Nations: Reform Initiatives Have Strengthened Operations, but Overall Objectives Have Not Yet Been Met. GAO/NSIAD-00-150, Washington, D.C.; May 10, 2000.

GAO's Mission	The Government Accountability Office, the audit, evaluation, and investigative arm of Congress, exists to support Congress in meeting its constitutional responsibilities and to help improve the performance and accountability of the federal government for the American people. GAO examines the use of public funds; evaluates federal programs and policies; and provides analyses, recommendations, and other assistance to help Congress make informed oversight, policy, and funding decisions. GAO's commitment to good government is reflected in its core values of accountability, integrity, and reliability.
Obtaining Copies of GAO Reports and Testimony	The fastest and easiest way to obtain copies of GAO documents at no cost is through GAO's website (www.gao.gov). Each weekday afternoon, GAO posts on its website newly released reports, testimony, and correspondence. To have GAO e-mail you a list of newly posted products, go to www.gao.gov and select "E-mail Updates."
Order by Phone	The price of each GAO publication reflects GAO's actual cost of production and distribution and depends on the number of pages in the publication and whether the publication is printed in color or black and white. Pricing and ordering information is posted on GAO's website, http://www.gao.gov/ordering.htm. Place orders by calling (202) 512-6000, toll free (866) 801-7077, or TDD (202) 512-2537. Orders may be paid for using American Express, Discover Card, MasterCard, Visa, check, or money order. Call for additional information.
Connect with GAO	Connect with GAO on Facebook, Flickr, Twitter, and YouTube. Subscribe to our RSS Feeds or E-mail Updates. Listen to our Podcasts. Visit GAO on the web at www.gao.gov.
To Report Fraud, Waste, and Abuse in Federal Programs	Contact: Website: www.gao.gov/fraudnet/fraudnet.htm E-mail: fraudnet@gao.gov Automated answering system: (800) 424-5454 or (202) 512-7470
Congressional Relations	Katherine Siggerud, Managing Director, siggerudk@gao.gov, (202) 512-4400, U.S. Government Accountability Office, 441 G Street NW, Room 7125, Washington, DC 20548
Public Affairs	Chuck Young, Managing Director, youngc1@gao.gov, (202) 512-4800 U.S. Government Accountability Office, 441 G Street NW, Room 7149 Washington, DC 20548

www.ingramcontent.com/pod-product-compliance
Lightning Source LLC
Chambersburg PA
CBHW080341290526
45791CB00009BA/2692